Essential Spanish for Pharmacists

Second Edition

Essential Spanish for Pharmacists

Second Edition

Glenn L. Kisch, PharmD
Owner, The Medicine Shoppe
Speedway, Indiana

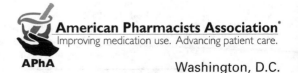

American Pharmacists Association®
Improving medication use. Advancing patient care.

APhA

Washington, D.C.

Managing Editor: Julian I. Graubart

Graphic and Cover Designer: Mary Jane Hickey

Proofreader: Suzanne Peake

© 2005 by the American Pharmacists Association

Published by the American Pharmacists Association, 2215 Constitution Avenue, N.W., Washington, DC 20037-2985 (http://www.aphanet.org)

APhA was founded in 1852 as the American Pharmaceutical Association.

To comment on this booklet via e-mail, send your message to the publisher at aphabooks@aphanet.org.

Library of Congress Cataloging-in-Publication Data
Kisch, Glenn L.
   Essential Spanish for pharmacists / Glenn L. Kisch. -- 2nd ed.
       p. ; cm.
   Text in English and Spanish.
   ISBN 1-58212-079-X
   1. Spanish language--Conversation and phrase books (for medical personnel)   I. American Pharmacists Association.   II. Title.
   [DNLM: 1. Pharmacy--Terminology--English.   2. Pharmacy
--Terminology--Spanish.   QV 715 K61e 2005]
PC4120.M3K57 2005
468.3'421'024615--dc22
                                                      2005017492

Contents

Acknowledgments

The author gratefully acknowledges the assistance of Julie Feest, PharmD, for her help in compiling the book's phrases and Michael Vance, PhD, for his help in reviewing the Spanish phraseology.

The publisher gratefully acknowledges the assistance of Magaly Rodriguez de Bittner, PharmD, BCPS, Enid Morales, PharmD, and Emmanuel Yentumi, who served as reviewers.

Initial Patient Encounter

Initial Patient Encounter

Greetings

English	Spanish	Pronunciation
Good morning	Buenos días	BWAIN-ohs DEE-ahs
Good afternoon	Buenas tardes	BWAIN-ahs TAHR-dais
Good evening	Buenas noches	BWAIN-ahs NOH-chais

Departures

English	Spanish	Pronunciation
Good-bye	Adiós	ah-dee-OHS
So long	Hasta luego	AH-stah lu-AI-go
Good night	Buenas noches	BWAIN-ahs NOH-chais
See you tomorrow.	Hasta mañana.	AH-stah mahn-YAHN-ah

Expressions of Courtesy

English	Spanish	Pronunciation
Please	Por favor	por fah-VOR
Thank you	Gracias	GRAH-see-ahs
You are welcome	De nada	dai NAH-dah
I beg your pardon.	Disculpe; perdón	dihs-KOOL-pai; pair-DOHN
Yes, sir	Sí, señor	see sen-YOR
No, sir	No, señor	no sen-YOR
Yes, madam	Sí, señora	see sen-YOR-ah
No, madam	No, señora	no sen-YOR-ah
Yes, miss	Sí, señorita	see se-nyo-REE-tah
No, miss	No, señorita	no se-nyo-REE-tah
With your permission	Con su permiso; con permiso; permiso	kon soo pair-MEE-so
You are very kind.	Usted es muy amable.	oos-TEHD ehs MOO-ey ah-MAHB-lai

Expressions of Courtesy (continued)

English	Spanish	Pronunciation
One moment, please.	Espere un momento, por favor.	eh-SPAIR-ai oon mo-MEN-toh por fah-VOR
I am grateful.	Le estoy muy agradecido; Estoy muy agredecido.	lai es-TOY MOO-ey ah-gra-deh-SEE-doh; es-TOY MOO-ey ah-grah-deh-SEE-doh
I am sorry.	Lo siento.	loh see-EN-to
How are you? How are you doing?	¿Cómo está usted? ¿Cómo está?	KOH-moh eh-STAH oos-TEHD; KOH-moh eh-STAH
Very well, thank you.	Muy bien, gracias.	MOO-ey bee-EN GRAH-see-ahs
May I help you?	¿En que puedo ayudarle? ¿Puedo ayudarle?	en kai PWAI-doh ai-yoo-DAHR-lai; PWAI-doh ai-yoo-DAHR-lai
What do you wish?	¿Que desea usted? ¿Desea algo?	kai deh-SAI-ah oos-TEHD; deh-SAI-ah AHL-go

Other Useful Expressions

English	Spanish	Pronunciation
What's happening?	¿Que pasa? ¿Qué hay de nuevo?	kai PAH-sah; kai AI dai noo-AI-voh
Do you speak English?	¿Habla usted inglés?	AH-blah oos-TEHD in-GLAIS
Yes, a little.	Sí, un poco; Sí, un poquito.	see oon POH-coh; see oon poh-KEE-toh
I speak a little Spanish.	Hablo un poco de español; Hablo un poquito de español; Hablo poquito español.	AH-bloh oon POH-koh dai ehs-pah-NYOL; AH-bloh oon poh-KEE-toh dai ehs-pah-NYOL; AH-bloh poh-KEE-toh ehs-pah-NYOL
Can you get an interpreter (a translator)?	¿Puede conseguir un intérprete (un traductor)?	PWAI-dai kon-seh-GEER oon in-TAIR-preh-tai (tra-duhk-TOR)
Do you understand (me)?	¿(Me) Entiende? ¿(Me) Comprende?	(mai) EN-tee-EN-dai; (mai) kom-PREN-dai
I (do not) understand.	Yo (no) comprendo; Yo (no) entiendo.	yoh (no) kom-PREN-doh; yoh (no) EN-tee-EN-doh

Other Useful Expressions (continued)

English	Spanish	Pronunciation
Of course	Sí, como no; Desde luego	see KOH-moh no; DEHS-dai loo-AI-goh
Speak slower, please.	Hable más despacio, por favor; Hable más de espacio, por favor.	ah-BLAI mahs dehs-PAH-see-oh, por fah-VOR; ah-BLAI mahs dai ehs-PAH-see-oh, por fah-VOR
Please repeat.	Repita por favor.	reh-PEE-tah por fah-VOR
Again	Otra vez	OH-trah vais
Do you know?	¿Sabe usted?	SAH-bai oos-TEHD
How do you say it?	¿Cómo se dice?	KOH-moh sai DEE-sai
How do you write it?	¿Cómo se escribe?	KOH-moh sai eh-SCREE-bai
You require a prescription.	Usted necesita una receta (del médico).	oos-TEHD neh-seh-SEE-tah OO-nah reh-SEH-tah (del MEH-dih-koh)
Can you prepare this prescription?	¿Puede usted preparar esta receta?	PWAI-dai oos-TEHD preh-pah-RARH EHS-tah reh-SEH-tah

Other Useful Expressions (continued)

English	Spanish	Pronunciation
Yes, we can.	Sí, podemos; Desde luego.	see poh-DAI-mohs; DAIS-dai loo-AI-go
This medication can't be obtained in the U.S.	Esta medicina no se puede conseguir en los Estados Unidos.	EHS-tah meh-dih-SEE-nah no sai PWAI-dai kon-sai-GEER en lohs es-TAH-dohs oo-NEE-dohs

Patient Data Collection

Patient Data Collection
General Information

English	Spanish	Pronunciation
What is your name?	¿Cómo se llama?	KOH-moh sai YAH-mah
My name is	Me llamo ____ ; Mi nombre es ____.	mai YAH-moh; mee NOHM-brai ehs
How old are you?	¿Qué edad tiene usted? ¿Cuántos años tiene usted? ¿Cuántos años tiene?	Kai ai-DAHD TEE-EN-ai oos-TEHD; KWAHN-tos AHN-yos TEE-EN-ai oos-TEHD; KWAHN-tos AHN-yos TEE-EN-ai
How old is the patient?	¿Cuál es la edad del paciente? ¿Cuántos años tiene el paciente?	kwahl ehs lah ai-DAHD dehl pah-see-EN-tai; KWAHN-tos AHN-yos TEE-EN-ai ehl pah-see-EN-tai
Birthdate	Fecha de nacimiento	FAI-cha dai nah-see-MEE-EN-to
Where do you live?	¿Dónde vive? ¿dónde vive usted?	DON-dai VEE-vai; DON-dai VEE-vai oos-TEHD
Give me your address.	Deme su dirección.	DAI-mai soo dee-rehk-see-OHN

General Information (continued)

English	Spanish	Pronunciation
What is your telephone number?	¿Cuál es el número de su teléfono?	kwahl ehs ehl NOO-mair-oh dai soo teh-LEH-fo-no
What is the telephone number?	¿Cuál es el número de teléfono?	kwahl ehs ehl NOO-mair-oh dai teh-LEH-fo-no
Please write it.	Hágame el favor de escribirlo.	AH-gah-me ehl fah-VOR dai ehs-kree-BEER-loh
Who is this prescription for?	¿Para quién es la receta?	PAH-rah KEE-en ehs lah reh-SEH-tah

Insurance Information

English	Spanish	Pronunciation
Do you receive Medicare or Medicaid?	¿Recibe usted Medicare o Medicaid?	RAI-see-bai oos-TEHD Medicare oh Medicaid
I need to see your latest insurance card.	Necesito ver su tarjeta de seguro médico más reciente.	neh-seh-SEE-toh vair soo tahr-HAI-tah dai sai-GOO-roh MEH-dee-koh MAS rai-see-EHN-tai
Do you have your identification card?	¿Tiene su tarjeta de identificación?	TEE-EN-ai soo tahr-HAI-tah dai ih-den-tih-fih-kah-see-OHN

Physician Information

English	Spanish	Pronunciation
What is your doctor's name and telephone number?	¿Cómo se llama su médico y cuál es el número de teléfono?	KOH-moh sai YAH-mah soo MEH-dee-koh ee kwahl ehs ehl NOO-mair-oh dai teh-LEH-fo-no
I will telephone the doctor for a prescription.	Yo llamaré al médico para la receta.	yoh yah-mah-RAI ahl MEH-dee-koh PAH-rah lah reh-SEH-tah
I will telephone the doctor for authorization to renew this prescription.	Yo llamaré al médico para que autorice la repetición de esta receta.	yoh yah-mah-RAI ahl MEH-dee-koh PAH-rah kai au-toh-RIH-sai lah reh-peh-tih-see-OHN dai EHS-tah reh-SEH-tah

Medication History

English	Spanish	Pronunciation
What medications are you taking at present?	¿Qué medicinas toma actualmente?	kai meh-dee-SEE-nahs TOH-mah ahk-tual-men-TAI
For how long?	¿Por cuánto tiempo?	por KWAN-toh tee-EM-poh
Are you using OTC medications?	¿Está usted tomando medicinas sin receta médica?	ehs-TAH oos-TEHD toh-MAHN-doh meh-dee-SIH-nahs seen reh-SEH-tah MEH-dee-kah

English	Spanish	Pronunciation
Are you using herbal products/home remedies?	¿Está usando productos naturales remedios caseros?	ehs-TAH oo-SAHN-doh proh-DUHK-tohs nah-too-RAH-lais reh-MAI-dee-ohs cah-SAI-rohs
What is your weight now?	¿Cuál es su peso actual? ¿Cuánto pesa actualmente?	kwahl ehs soo PAI-so ahk-TUAL; KWAN-toh PAI-sah ahk-tual-MEN-tai
What is your height?	¿Cuánto mide usted? ¿Cuánto mide?	KWAN-toh MEE-dai oos-TEHD; KWAN-toh MEE-dai
Do you smoke?	¿Usted fuma?	oos-TEHD FOO-mah
cigarettes	cigarillos	sih-gahr-REE-yohs
cigars	cigarros	sih-GAHR-rohs
pipe	pipa	PEE-pah
marijuana	marihuana	mah-rih-hoo-AN-ah
I have never smoked.	No he fumado nunca.	no hai foo-MAH-doh NOON-kah
Have you ever smoked?	¿Ha fumado usted alguna vez? ¿Ha fumado usted en el pasado?	hah foo-MAH-doh oos-TEHD ahl-GOO-nah vais; hah foo-MAH-doh oos-TEHD ehn ehl pah-SAH-doh

Medication History (continued)

English	Spanish	Pronunciation
I gave it up.	He dejado de fumar.	hai dai-HA-doh dai foo-MAR
Have you given up smoking?	¿Dejó usted de fumar?	dai-HO oos-TEHD dai foo-MAR
Do you drink alcohol?	¿Usted bebe alcohol? ¿Usted bebe bebidas alcohólicas?	oos-TEHD BAI-bai ahl-koh-HOL; oos-TEHD BAI-bai bai-BEE-dahs ahl-koh-HOH-lee-kahs
wine	vino	VEE-noh
rum	ron	rohn
hard liquor	bebidas fuertes	bai-BEE-dahs FWAIR-tais
beer	cerveza	ser-VAI-sah
What medications are you allergic to?	¿A qué medicinas es alérgico usted?	ah KAI me-dee-SEE-nahs ehs ah-LAIR-hee-koh oos-TEHD
none	ninguna	neen-GOO-nah
aspirin	aspirina	ahs-pee-REE-nah
codeine	codeína	koh-dai-EE-nah
novocaine	novocaína	noh-voh-ka-EE-nah

Medication History (continued)

English	Spanish	Pronunciation
penicillin	penicilina	pe-ni-sih-LEE-nah
sulfa	las sulfas	las SOOL-fahs
tetanus	tétano	TEH-ta-noh
xylocaine	xilocaína	zi-loh-ka-EE-nah

Section 3

Patient Consultation Directions

Patient Consultation Directions
Prescription Dispensing Information

English	Spanish	Pronunciation
One moment, please.	Espere un momento, por favor.	ehs-PAI-rai oon mo-MEN-to por fah-VOR
When will it be ready?	¿Cuándo estará lista?	KWAN-do ehs-ta-RAH LIHS-tah
Please take a seat.	Siéntese por favor; Tome asiento, por favor.	see-EHN-teh-sai por fah-VOR; TOH-mai ah-see-EHN-to por fah-VOR
We will have it ready as soon as possible.	Estará listo lo más pronto posible; Su receta estará lista lo más pronto posible.	es-stah-RAH LIHS-toh loh MAHS PRON-to poh-SEE-blai; Soo reh-SEH-tah es-tah-RAH LIHS-tah loh MAHS PRON-to poh-SEE-blai
It will take _____ minutes.	Esta receta demorará _____ minutos.	ES-tah reh-SEH-tah dai-mor-rah-RAH __ mi-NOO-tohs
Please come back at_____ .	Vuelva a las _____ por favor.	VWEL-vah ah lahs ___ por fah-VOR
Please come back in _____ minutes.	Vuelva en _____ minutos por favor.	VWEL-vah ehn ___ mi-NOO-tohs por fah-VOR

Prescription Dispensing Information (continued)

English	Spanish	Pronunciation
Please come back in a half hour.	Vuelva en media hora por favor.	VWEL-vah ehn MAI-dee-ah OH-rah por fah-VOR
We do not stock the item.	No tenemos el producto disponible; No lo tenemos a mano.	no tai-NE-mohs ehl proh-DUHK-to DIHS-po-NEE-blai; no lo tai-NE-mohs ah MAH-no
We will order it for you.	Se lo ordenaremos.	sai lo or-deh-nah-RAI-mohs
It will take ___ days to receive it.	Tardará ___ días para recibirlo.	tahr-dah-RAH ___ DEE-ahs PAH-rah rai-see-BEER-loh

Duration

English	Spanish	Pronunciation
for ___ week(s)	por ___ semana(s)	por ___ sai-MAH-nah(s)
for ___ days	por ___ días	por ___ DEE-ahs
for ___ days, then discontinue	por ___ días, luego deje de tomarlo	por ___ DEE-ahs, loo-AI-go DAI-hai dai toh-MAR-lo
until finished	hasta que se termine	AH-stah kai sai tair-MEE-nai

Administration Instructions

(see also Commonly Used Verbs, page 44 in Glossary)

English	Spanish	Pronunciation
Take one tablet every day.	Tome una tableta (una pastilla) cada día.	TOH-mai OO-nah tah-BLEH-tah (OO-nah pahs-TEE-yah) CAH-dah DEE-ah
Take two capsules three times a day.	Tome dos cápsulas tres veces al día.	TOH-mai dohs KAHP-soo-lahs trehs VAI-sais ahl DEE-ah
Take one or two tablets every four hours as needed for pain.	Tome una o dos tabletas cada cuatro horas si la necesita para el dolor.	TOH-mai OO-nah oh dohs tah-BLEH-tas CAH-dah KWAH-tro OH-rahs see lah neh-seh-SEE-tah PAH-rah ehl doh-LOHR
Take one tablet three times daily with meals.	Tome una tableta tres veces al día con las comidas.	TOH-mai OO-nah tah-BLEH-tah trehs VAI-sais ahl DEE-ah kon lahs koh-MEE-dahs
Take one capsule at bedtime as needed for sleep.	Tome una cápsula al acostarse si la necesita para dormir.	TOH-mai OO-nah KAHP-soo-lah ahl ah-kohs-TAHR-sai see lah neh-seh-SEE-tah PAH-rah dor-MEER
Take ½ teaspoonful three times a day.	Tome media cucharadita tres veces al día.	TOH-mai MAI-dee-ah koo-cha-rah-DEE-tah trehs VAI-sais ahl DEE-ah

English	Spanish	Pronunciation
Take one tea-spoonful every four hours as needed for fever.	Tome una cucharadita cada cuatro horas si la necesita para la fiebre.	TOH-mai OO-nah koo-cha-rah-DEE-tah CAH-dah KWAH-tro OH-rahs see lah neh-seh-SEE-tah PAH-rah lah fee-AI-brai
Take one tablet four times a day before (with, after) meals and at bedtime.	Tome una pastilla cuatro veces al día, antes (con, después) de la comida y al acostarse.	TOH-mai OO-nah pahs-TEE-yah KWAH-tro VAI-sais ahl DEE-ah, AHN-tais (kon, dehs-poo-AIS) dai lah koh-MEE-dah ee ahl ah-kohs-TAHR-sai
Remove wrapping and insert one suppository rectally/vaginally.	Quite la envoltura e insértese un supositorio rectalmente/vaginalmente.	KEE-tai lah en-vol-TOO-rah ee in-SAIR-tai-sai oon soo-pah-see-TOH-ree-oh rehk-TAHL-mehn-tai/vah-hee-NAHL-mehn-tai
Insert one applicatorful vaginally.	Llene el aplicador e insérteselo vaginalmente.	YAI-nai ehl ah-plee-kah-DOR ee in-SAIR-tai-seh-lo vah-hee-NAHL-mehn-tai
Instill ___ drops in affected eye(s).	Echese ___ gota(s) en el (los) ojo(s) afectado(s).	eh-CHAI-sai ___ goh-TAH(S) ehn ehl (lohs) OH-ho(s) ah-fehk-TAH-doh(s)

Administration Instructions (continued)

English	Spanish	Pronunciation
Inject ____ units subcutaneously.	Inyectar ____ unidades debajo de la piel (subcutáneamente).	in-yehk-TAHR ____ oo-nee-DAH-dais dai-BAH-ho dai lah PEE-el (suhb-coo-TAH-nai-ah-mehn-tai)
Apply externally ____ times a day.	Aplíque externamente____ veces al día.	ah-PLEE-kai ehks-TER-nah-mehn-tai ____ VAI-sais ahl DEE-ah
Apply to skin sparingly.	Aplíque una capa delgada sobre la piel; Aplíque una capa lígera.	ah-PLEE-kai OO-nah CAH-pah dehl-GAH-dah soh-BRAI lah pee-EL; ah-PLEE-kai OO-nah CAH-pah lee-HAIR-rah
Apply to painful parts.	Aplíque en las partes adoloridas.	ah-PLEE-kai ehn lahs PAHR-tais ah-doh-loh-REE-dahs
Apply on affected parts.	Aplíque en partes afectadas.	ah-PLEE-kai ehn PAHR-tais ah-fek-TAH-dahs
Apply to affected area(s).	Aplíque en el (las) área(s) afectada(s).	ah-PLEE-kai ehn ehl (lahs) AH-rai-ah(s) ah-fek-TAH-dah(s)
Chew____tablets every day.	Mastique____ tableta(s) cada día.	mahs-TEE-kai ____ tah-BLEH-tah(s) CAH-dah DEE-ah

Administration Instructions (continued)

English	Spanish	Pronunciation
Do not chew; swallow whole.	No las mastique; tráguelas enteras.	no lahs mahs-TEE-kai; TRAH-gai-lahs ehn-TAIR-rahs
Shake well before using.	Agítese bien antes de usarse; Agite bien antes de usarse.	ah-HEE-tai-sai BEE-ehn AHN-tais dai oo-SAHR-sai; ah-HEE-tai BEE-ehn AHN-tais dai oo-SAHR-sai
Use as directed by the physician.	Utilice como le indicó el médico.	oo-tee-LEE-sai KOH-moh lai in-dee-KOH ehl MEH-dee-koh
Consult your physician.	Consulte a su médico.	kon-SOOL-tai ah soo MEH-dee-koh
For external use	Para uso externo	PAH-rah oo-soh ehks-TAIR-noh
Use as mouthwash.	Use para enjuagarse la boca.	oo-sai PAH-rah en-hwa-GAHR-sai lah BOH-cah
Do not take at same time as other medicines.	No tome este medicamento al mismo tiempo que otras medicinas.	no TOH-mai EHS-tai meh-dee-cah-MEHN-toh ahl MEES-moh tee-EHM-poh kai OH-trahs meh-dee-SEE-nahs
Take medication on an empty stomach.	Tome esta medicina con el estómago vació.	TOH-mai EHS-tah meh-dee-SEE-nah kon ehl ehs-TOH-mah-go vah-SEE-oh

English	Spanish	Pronunciation
Do not drink alcoholic beverages while taking this medicine.	No tome bebidas alcohólicas mientras toma esta medicina.	no TOH-mai bai-BEE-dahs ahl-koh-HOH-lee-kahs mee-EN-trahs TOH-mah EHS-tah meh-dee-SEE-nah
Take this medication with plenty of water.	Tome este medicamento con mucha agua.	TOH-mai EHS-tai meh-dee-kah-MEHN-to kon MOO-chah AH-gwah
Do not drink milk or milk products while taking this medication.	No tome leche o productos lácteos mientras toma esta medicina.	no TOH-mai LEH-chai o proh-DOOK-tohs LAHK-tai-ohs mee-EN-trahs TOH-mah EHS-tah meh-dee-SEE-nah
Do not drive or operate heavy machinery while taking this medication.	No maneje u opere maquinaria peligrosa mientras esté tomando este medicamento.	no mah-NAI-hai oo oh-PAIR-rai mah-kee-NAH-ree-ah peh-lee-GROH-sah mee-EN-trahs ehs-TAI toh-MAHN-doh EHS-tai meh-dee-kah-MEHN-toh.
Consult your doctor if you are pregnant or nursing.	Consulte a su médico si está embarazada o lactando.	kon-SOOL-tai ah soo MEH-dee-koh see ehs-TAH em-bah-ra-SAH-dah oh lahk-TAHN-doh

Administration Instructions (continued)

English	Spanish	Pronunciation
Do not use this medication if pregnant or nursing.	No use este medicamento si está embarazada o lactando.	no OO-sai EHS-tai meh-dee-kah-MEHN-toh see ehs-TAH em-bah-rah-SAH-dah oh lahk-TAHN-doh
Avoid sunlight while taking this medication.	Evite exponerse al sol mientras esté usando este medicamento.	ai-VEE-tai ehks-po-NAIR-sai ahl sohl mee-EN-trahs ehs-TAI oo-SAHN-doh EH-stai meh-dee-kah-MEHN-toh

Side Effects

English	Spanish	Pronunciation
may cause...	puede causar...	PWAI-dai kau-SAHR
bleeding	sangrado	sahn-GRAH-doh
dizziness	mareos	mah-RAI-ohs
increase/decrease of appetite	aumento/diminución del apetito	ou-MEN-toh/dee-mee-noo-see-OHN dehl ah-peh-TEE-toh
photosensitivity	sensibilidad a la luz solar	sen-see-bee-LEE-dahd ah lah LOOS soh-LAHR

Side Effects (continued)

English	Spanish	Pronunciation
sleepiness	sueño	SWAIN-yo
tremor	tremblor	trehm-BLOHR
weight gain	aumeto de peso	ou-MEN-toh dai PAI-soh

Refill Information

English	Spanish	Pronunciation
Return the bottle to us.	Traíganos el frasco.	TRAH-EE-gah-nos ehl FRAHS-coh
This prescription may not be repeated.	Esta receta no se puede repetir.	EHS-tah reh-SEH-tah no sai PWAI-dai reh-pai-TEER
This prescription may be repeated once.	Esta receta se puede repetir una vez más.	EHS-tah reh-SEH-tah sai PWAI-dai reh-pai-TEER OO-nah vais MAHS
This prescription may be repeated twice.	Esta receta se puede repetir dos veces más.	EHS-tah reh-SEH-tah sai PWAI-dai reh-pai-TEER dohs VAI-sais MAHS

Storage

English	Spanish	Pronunciation
Keep in the refrigerator.	Guárdelo en la nevera; Guárdelo en el refrigerador; Manténgase en la nevera.	GWAHR-day-loh ehn lah nai-VAI-rah; GWAHR-day-loh ehn ehl rai-frih-hair-rah-DOHR; man-TEN-gah-sai ehn lah nai-VAI-rah
Do not refrigerate.	No refrigere; No necesita refrigerarse.	no rai-frih-HAIR-rai; no neh-seh-SEE-tah rai-frih-hair-RAHR-sai
Keep this and all medicines out of reach of children.	Mantenga ésta y todas las medicinas fuera del alcance de los niños.	man-TEN-gah EHS-tah ee TOH-dahs lahs meh-dee-SEE-nahs FWAI-rah dehl ahl-KAHN-sai dai lohs NEE-nyohs
Keep tightly closed.	Manténgase bien cerrado.	man-TEN-gah-sai BEE-en sair-RAH-do
Store in a cool, dry place.	Almacéne en un sitio fresco y seco; Guarde en un sitio fresco y seco.	ahl-mah-SEH-nai ehn oon SEE-tee-oh FREHS-koh ee SAI-koh; GWAHR-dai ehn oon SEE-tee-oh FREHS-koh ee SAI-koh
Store away from heat and sunlight.	Guarde fuera del calor y de la luz del sol.	GWAHR-dai FWAI-rah dehl kah-LOHR ee dai lah loos dehl sohl

Storage (continued)

English	Spanish	Pronunciation
May be kept at room temperature for 14 days without loss of potency.	Puede mantenerse a temperatura ambiente por catorce días sin perder la potencia.	PWAI-dai man-teh-NAIR-sai ah tehm-pair-rah-TOO-rah ahm-BEE-EN-tai por kah-TOR-sai DEE-ahs seen pair-DAIR lah poh-TEHN-see-ah
Keep these tablets in original container to prevent loss of potency.	Conserve estas tabletas en su envase original para evitar que pierdan su potencia.	kon-SAIR-vai EHS-tahs tah-BLEH-tahs ehn soo ehn-VAH-sai or-reeh-hih-NAHL PAH-rah ai-vee-TAHR kai pee-AIR-dan soo poh-TEHN-see-ah
Do not use after this date.	No use después de esta fecha.	no OO-sai des-poo-AIS dai EHS-tah FAI-cha

Use

English	Spanish	Pronunciation
for allergy	para la alergia	PAH-rah lah ah-LAIR-hee-ah
for anxiety	para la ansiedad; para los nervios	PAH-rah lah ahn-see-ai-DAHD; PAH-rah lohs NAIR-vee-ohs

English	Spanish	Pronunciation
for arrhythmias	para aritmias (palpitaciones)	PAH-rah ah-REET-mee-ahs pahl-pee-tah-see-OH-nais
for arthritis	para la artritis	PAH-rah lah ahr-TREE-tis
for asthma	para el asma	PAH-rah ehl AHS-mah
for backache	para el dolor de espalda	PAH-rah ehl doh-LOHR dai ehs-PAHL-da
for chest pain	para el dolor del pecho	PAH-rah ehl doh-LOHR dehl PAI-cho
for cold	para el catarro (para el resfriado)	PAH-rah ehl kah-TAHR-roh (PAH-rah ehl rehs-free-AH-doh)
for constipation	para el estreñimiento	PAH-rah ehl ehs-treh-nyee-mee-EHN-toh
for cough	para la tos	PAH-rah lah tohs
for cramps	Para los calambres; para los retortijones	PAH-rah lohs cah-LAHM-brais; PAH-rah lohs rai-tohr-tee-HOHN-ais
for depression	para la depresión	PAH-rah lah deh-preh-see-OHN

English	Spanish	Pronunciation
for diarrhea	para la diarrea	PAH-rah lah dee-ah-REE-ah
for dizziness	para los mareos	PAH-rah lohs mah-RAI-ohs
for earache	para el dolor de oído	PAH-rah ehl doh-LOHR dai oh-EE-doh
for edema	para el edema	PAH-rah ehl ai-DAI-mah
for fever	para la fiebre; la calentura	PAH-rah lah fee-AI-brai; lah kah-lehn-TOO-rah
for fungus	para el hongo	PAH-rah ehl ON-go
for headache	para el dolor de cabeza	PAH-rah ehl doh-LOHR dai kah-BAI-sah
for the heart	para el corazón	PAH-rah ehl koh-rah-SON
for high blood pressure	para la presión alta	PAH-rah lah preh-see-OHN AHL-tah
for infection	para la infección	PAH-rah lah in-feck-see-OHN
for inflammation	para la inflamación	PAH-rah lah in-flah-mah-see-OHN
for insomnia	para el insomnio	PAH-rah ehl in-SOM-nee-oh

English	Spanish	Pronunciation
for the kidneys	para los riñones	PAH-rah lohs ree-NYOH-nais
for lice	para los piojos	PAH-rah lohs pee-OH-hohs
for menstrual pain/cramps	para el dolor/calambres de la menstruación	PAH-rah ehl doh-LOHR/cah-LAHM-brais dai lah mehns-troo-ah-see-OHN
for motion sickness	para el mareo	PAH-rah ehl mar-RAI-oh
for nausea	para la náusea	PAH-rah lah NOW-sai-ah
for pain	para dolor/para el dolor	PAH-rah doh-LOHR/PAH-rah ehl doh-LOHR
for PMS	para el síndrome premenstrual	PAH-rah ehl SIN-droh-mai PRAI-mehns-troo-AHL
for shortness of breath	para la respiracción corta; para la dificultad al respirar	PAH-rah lah res-pee-rah-see-OHN KOHR-tah; PAH-rah lah dih-fih-kuhl-TAHD ahl rehs-pee-RAHR
for sleep	para dormir	PAH-rah dor-MEER
for sore throat	para el dolor de garganta	PAH-rah ehl DOH-lohr dai gahr-GAN-ta

English	Spanish	Pronunciation
for stomach pain	para el dolor de estómago	PAH-rah ehl doh-LOHR dai ehs-TOH-mah-go
for stuffy nose/runny nose	para la nariz tupida/gotereo nasal	PAH-rah lah nah-REES too-PEE-dah; goh-taih-RAI-oh nah-SAHL
for swelling	para la hinchazón	PAH-rah lah een-cha-SON
for ulcer(s)	para la úlcera(s)	PAH-rah lah(s) UHL-seh-rah(s)
for urine infection	para la infección de orina	PAH-rah lah in-fehk-see-OHN dai or-REE-nah

Glossary

Glossary

Days of the Week

English	Spanish	Pronunciation
Sunday	domingo	doh-MIN-goh
Monday	lunes	LOO-nais
Tuesday	martes	MAHR-tais
Wednesday	miércoles	mee-AIR-koh-lais
Thursday	jueves	HWAI-vais
Friday	viernes	vee-AIR-nais
Saturday	sábado	SAH-bah-doh

Numbers

English	Spanish	Pronunciation
none	ninguno	neen-GOO-no
zero (0)	cero	SAI-roh
one-quarter (¼)	un cuarto	oon KWAR-toh
one-half (½)	media; medio	MAI-dee-ah; MAI-dee-oh
three-quarters (¾)	tres cuartos	trehs KWAR-tohs
one (1)	una/uno	OO-nah/OO-no

Numbers (continued)

English	Spanish	Pronunciación
one and one-half (1½)	una y media	OO-nah ee MAI-dee-ah
two (2)	dos	dohs
three (3)	tres	trehs
four (4)	cuatro	KWAH-tro
five (5)	cinco	SEEN-ko
six (6)	seis	sais
seven (7)	siete	see-EH-tai
eight (8)	ocho	OH-cho
nine (9)	nueve	noo-AI-vai
ten (10)	diez	dee-AIS
eleven (11)	once	ON-sai
twelve (12)	doce	DOH-sai
thirteen (13)	trece	TREH-sai
fourteen (14)	catorce	kah-TOR-sai
fifteen (15)	quince	KEEN-sai
sixteen (16)	diez y seis; dieciséis	dee-ais ee SAIS

Numbers (continued)

English	Spanish	Pronunciation
English	*Spanish*	*Pronunciation*
seventeen (17)	diez y siete; diecisiete	dee-AIS ee see-EH-tai
eighteen (18)	diez y ocho; dieciocho	dee-AIS ee OH-cho
nineteen (19)	diez y nueve; diecinueve	dee-AIS ee noo-AI-vai
twenty (20)	veinte	VAIN-tai
twenty-one (21)	veintiuno/a	vain-tee-OO-noh/nah
thirty (30)	treinta	TRAIN-tah
forty (40)	cuarenta	kwah-REN-tah
fifty (50)	cincuenta	seen-KWEN-tah
sixty (60)	sesenta	seh-SEHN-tah
seventy (70)	setenta	seh-TEN-tah
eighty (80)	ochenta	oh-CHEN-tah
ninety (90)	noventa	noh-VEN-tah
one hundred (100)	cien	see-EHN
one hundred one (101)	ciento uno/a	see-EHN-toh OO-noh/nah

Numbers (continued)

English	Spanish	Pronunciation
two hundred (200)	dos cientos	dohs see-EHN-tohs
one thousand (1000)	mil	meel
nineteen fifty (1950)	mil novecientos cincuenta	meel noh-veh-see-EHN-tohs seen-KWEN-tah
nineteen ninety-nine (1999)	mil novecientos noventa y nueve	mee noh-veh-see-EHN-tohs noh-VEN-tah ee noo-AI-vai
two thousand (2000)	dos mil	dohs meel

Colors

English	Spanish	Pronunciation
black	negro	NAI-groh
blue	azul	ah-SOOL
brown	pardo; moreno	PAHR-doh; moh-RAI-noh
gray	gris	grees
green	verde	VAIR-dai
orange	anaranjado	ahn-ar-ahn-HA-doh

Colors (continued)

English	Spanish	Pronunciation
pink	rosa	ROH-sah
purple	purpúreo; violeta	pur-PU-rai-oh; vee-oh-LAI-tah
red	rojo	ROH-hoh
white	blanco	BLAHN-ko
yellow	amarillo	ah-mah-REE-yo

Relations

English	Spanish	Pronunciation
aunt	tía	TEE-ah
brother	hermano	air-MAH-noh
brother-in-law	cuñado	koo-NYAH-doh
cousin	primo, prima	PREE-moh, PREE-mah
daughter	hija	EE-ha
father	padre	PAH-drai
father-in-law	suegro	SWAI-gro

Relations (continued)

English	Spanish	Pronunciation
friend (male)	amigo	ah-MEE-go
friend (female)	amiga	ah-MEE-gah
granddaughter	nieta	nee-AI-ta
grandfather	abuelo	ah-BWAI-lo
grandmother	abuela	ah-BWAI-lah
grandson	nieto	nee-AI-toh
husband	esposo	ehs-POH-so
mother	madre	MAH-drai
mother-in-law	suegra	SWAI-grah
nephew	sobrino	soh-BREE-no
niece	sobrina	soh-BREE-nah
sister	hermana	air-MAH-nah
sister-in-law	cuñada	koo-NYAH-dah
son	hijo	EE-ho
uncle	tío	TEE-oh
wife	esposa	ehs-POH-sah

Parts of the Body

English	Spanish	Pronunciation
abdomen	el abdomen; la barriga	ehl ahb-DOH-men; lah bah-REE-gah
ankle	el tobillo	ehl toh-BEE-yoh
arm	el brazo	ehl BRAH-so
back	la espalda; el dorso	lah ehs-PAHL-dah; ehl DOR-soh
bone	el hueso	ehl HWAI-so
breasts	los senos	lohs SEH-nohs
buttocks	las nalgas; el trasero	lahs NAHL-gahs; ehl trah-SAI-roh
calf	la pantorrilla	lah pahn-toh-REE-yah
cheek	a mejilla	lah meh-HEE-yah
chest	el pecho	ehl PAI-cho
chin	la barbilla	lah bahr-BEE-yah
ear	el oído (inner); la oreja (outer)	ehl oh-EE-doh; lah oh-RAI-ha
elbow	el codo	ehl KOH-doh

Parts of the Body (continued)

English	Spanish	Pronunciation
eye	el ojo	ehl OH-ho
eyelid	el párpado	ehl PAHR-pah-doh
face	la cara	lah CAH-rah
fingers	los dedos de la mano	lohs DAI-dohs dai lah MAH-noh
foot/feet	el pie; los pies	ehl pee-AI; lohs pee-AIS
forehead	la frente	lah FREHN-tai
gums	las encías	lahs ehn-SEE-ahs
hair	el cabello; el pelo	ehl kah-BAI-yo; ehl PAI-loh
hand	la mano	lah MAH-noh
head	la cabeza	lah kah-BAI-sah
heart	el corazón	ehl koh-rah-SON
heel	el talón	ehl tah-LOHN
hip	la cadera	ah kah-DEH-rah
kidney	el riñón	ehl ree-NYON

Parts of the Body (continued)

English	Spanish	Pronunciation
knee	la rodilla	lah roh-DEE-yah
leg	la pierna	lah pee-AIR-nah
lip	el labio	ehl LAH-bee-oh
liver	el hígado	ehl ee-GAH-doh
mouth	la boca	lah BOH-kah
muscle	el músculo	ehl MOOS-koo-loh
nails	las uñas	lahs OO-nyahs
neck	el cuello	ehl KWAI-yo
nerve	el nervio	ehl NAIR-vee-oh
nose	la nariz	lah nah-REES
prostate	la próstata	lah PROHS-tah-tah
scalp	cuero cabelludo	koo-EH-roh kah-beh-YOO-doh
shoulders	los hombros	lohs OM-brohs
skin	la piel	lah PEE-el

Parts of the Body (continued)

English	Spanish	Pronunciation
stomach	el estómago	ehl ehs-TOH-mah-go
thigh	el muslo	ehl MOOS-lo
throat	la garganta	lah gahr-GAN-tah
toes	los dedos de los pies	lohs DAI-dohs dai lohs pee-AIS
tongue	la lengua	lah LAING-gwah
tonsils	las amígdalas	lahs ah-MIHG-dah-lahs
tooth/teeth	el diente/los dientes	ehl dee-EHN-tai/lohs dee-EHN-tais
vagina	la vagina	lah vah-HEE-nah
vertebra	la vértebra	lah VAIR-tai-brah
wrist	la muñeca	lah moo-NYAI-kah

Commonly Used Verbs

English	Spanish	Pronunciation
apply	aplique	ah-PLIH-kai
chew	mastique	mahs-TEE-kai
chew and swallow	mastique y trague	mahs-TEE-kai ee TRAH-gai
dilute	diluya	dee-LOO-yah
dissolve	disuelva	dih-SWAEL-vah
inject	inyecte	in-YEHK-tai
insert	inserte	ihn-SAIR-tai
instill	eche	EH-chai
mix	mezcle	MEHS-kle
place	coloque; ponga	koh-LOH-kai; POHN-gah
put	ponga	POHN-gah
rub	frote	FROH-tai
shampoo	champú	cham-POO
sprinkle	esparcir	ehs-pahr-SEER

Commonly Used Verbs (continued)

English	Spanish	Pronunciation
take	tome	TOH-mai
use	use	OO-sai

Measurements

English	Spanish	Pronunciation
applicatorful	aplicador lleno	ah-plee-kah-DOHR YAI-no
dropperful(s)	gotero(s) lleno(s)	goh-TAI-roh(s) YAI-no(s)
inch	pulgada	puhl-GAH-dah
milligrams	miligramos	mih-lih-GRAH-mos
milliliters	mililitros	mih-lih-LEE-trohs
ounce(s)	onza(s)	ON-sah(s)
tablespoonful(s)	cucharada(s)	koo-cha-RAH-dah(s)
teaspoonful(s)	cucharadita(s)	koo-cha-rah-DEE-tah(s)
units	unidades	OO-nee-DAH-dais

Dosage Forms

English	Spanish	Pronunciation
capsule(s)	cápsula(s)	KAHP-soo-lah(s)
cream	crema	KRAI-mah
drops	gota(s)	GOH-tah(s)
elixir	elíxir	eh-LEEK-sair
inhalation/spray inhaler	inhalación/inhalador	in-hah-lah-see-OHN/in-hah-lah-DOHR
injection	inyección	in-yehk-see-OHN
liquid	líquido	LIH-kee-doh
ointment	ungüento; untura	uhn-GWEN-toh; uhn-TOO-rah
patch	parcho	PAHR-cho
pill	píldora; pastilla	PIHL-doh-rah; pahs-TEE-yah
powder	polvo	POHL-voh
suppository	supositorio	soo-poh-see-TOH-ree-oh

Dosage Forms (continued)

English	Spanish	Pronunciation
tablet(s)	tableta(s)	tah-BLEH-tah(s)
troche	pastilla; tableta para chupar	pahs-TEE-YAH; tah-BLEH-tah PAH-rah chu-PAHR

Drug Administration Routes

otic

English	Spanish	Pronunciation
in the left ear	en el oído (oreja) izquierdo	ehn ehl oh-EE-doh (oh-RAI-ha) ihs-kee-AIR-doh
in the right ear	en el oído (oreja) derecho	ehn ehl oh-EE-doh (oh-RAI-ha) deh-RAI-cho
in each ear	en cada oído (oreja)	ehn CAH-dah oh-EE-doh (oh-RAI-ha)
in both ears	en ambos oídos	ehn AHM-bohs oh-EE-dohs

ophthalmic

English	Spanish	Pronunciation
in affected eye(s)	en el (los) ojo(s) afectado(s)	ehn ehl (lohs) OH-ho(s) ah-fek-TAH-doh(s)
in the left eye	en el ojo izquierdo	ehn ehl OH-ho ihs-kee-AIR-doh
in the right eye	en el ojo derecho	ehn ehl OH-ho deh-RAI-cho
in each eye	en cada ojo	ehn CAH-dah OH-ho
in both eyes	en ambos ojos	ehn AHM-bohs OH-hos

oral

English	Spanish	Pronunciation
buccally (between gum and cheek)	entre la enciá y la mejilla	ehn-TRAI lah ehn-SEE-ah ee lah meh-HEE-yah
sublingual; under the tongue	sublingual; debajo de la lengua	suhb-LEEN-gwahl; dai-BAH-hoh dai lah LAIN-gwah

Drug Administration Routes (continued)

nasal

English	Spanish	Pronunciation
in each nostril	en cada fosa nasal	ehn CAH-dah FOH-sah nah-SAHL

topical and subcutaneous

English	Spanish	Pronunciation
externally	externamente	ehks-TER-nah-mehn-tai
to skin	sobre la piel; en la piel	soh-BRAI lah pee-EL; ehn lah PEE-el
subcutaneously	debajo de la piel; subcutánea	dai-BAH-ho dai lah pee-EL; suhb-koo-TAH-nai-ah
subcutaneous injection	inyección subcutánea	in-yehk-see-OHN suhb-koo-TAH-nai-ah

vaginal

English	Spanish	Pronunciation
as a douche	para lavado; lavado vaginal; ducha vaginal	PAH-rah lah-VAH-doh; lah-VAH-doh vah-hee-NAHL; DOO-cha vah-hee-NAHL
vaginally	vaginalmente; en la vagina	vah-hee-NAHL-mehn-tai; ehn lah vah-HEE-nah

Drug Administration Routes (continued)

other

English	Spanish	Pronunciation
intramuscular injection	inyección intramuscular	in-yehk-see-OHN ihn-trah-moos-koo-LAHR
intravenous	intravenosa	ihn-trah-veh-NOH-sah
rectally	rectalmente; en el recto	rehk-TAHL-mehn-tai; ehn ehl RAIK-to

Frequency

English	Spanish	Pronunciation
daily	cada día; diariamente; una vez al día; diario	CAH-dah DEE-ah; dee-AH-riah-mehn-tai; OO-nah vais ahl DEE-ah; dee-AH-ree-oh.
___ times a day	___ veces al dia	___ vai-SAIS ahl DEE-ah
bid	dos veces al día	dohs VAI-sais alh DEE-ah
tid	tres veces al día	trehs VAI-sais ahl DEE-ah
qid	cuatro veces al día	KWAH-tro VAI-sais ahl DEE-ah

Frequency (continued)

English	Spanish	Pronunciation
every second day; every other day; alternate days	un día si y otro no; día de por medio; un día si y un día no	oon DEE-ah see ee OH-troh no; DEE-ah dai por MAI-dee-oh; oon DEE-ah see ee oon DEE-ah no
as needed	si la necesita; como sea necesario	see lah neh-seh-SEE-tah; COH-moh SAI-ah neh-seh-SAH-ree-oh
every ___ hours	cada ___ horas	CAH-dah ___ OH-rahs
if necessary	si es necesario	see ehs neh-seh-SAH-ree-oh
if necessary, repeat in __ hours	si es necesario, repítalo en __ horas	see ehs neh-seh-SAH-ree-oh, rai-PEE-tah-loh ehn __ OH-rahs

Time of Day

English	Spanish	Pronunciation
daily in the morning	cada día, por la mañana	CAH-dah DEE-ah, por lah mah-NYA-nah
at noon	al medio día	ahl MAI-dee-oh DEE-ah
in the afternoon	en la tarde	ehn lah TAHR-dai

Time of Day (continued)

English	Spanish	Pronunciation
daily in the evening	cada día, por la noche	CAH-dah DEE-ah, por lah NOH-chai
before retiring	antes de acostarse	AHN-tais dai ah-kohs-TAHR-sai
at bedtime	al acostarse	Ahl ah-kohs-TAHR-sai
while awake	mientras esté despierto	mee-EN-trahs ehs-TAI dais-pee-AIR-toh

Meals

English	Spanish	Pronunciation
before meals	antes de las comidas	AHN-tais dai lahs koh-MEE-dahs
after meals	después de las comidas	dehs-poo-EHS dai lahs koh-MEE-dahs
with meals	con las comidas	kon lahs koh-MEE-dahs
with breakfast	con el desayuno	kon ehl dehs-ah-YOO-noh
with lunch	con el almuerzo	kon ehl ahl-MWAIR-so
with supper (dinner)	con la cena (comida)	kon lah SAI-nah (koh-MEE-dah)

Meals (continued)

English	Spanish	Pronunciation
between meals	entre comidas	EHN-trai koh-MEE-dahs
fasting	en ayunas	ehn ai-YOO-nahs
on an empty stomach	con el estómago vacío	kon ehl es-TOH-mah-go vah-SEE-oh
in a quart (pint) of hot/cold/boiling/ warm water	en un cuarto (pinta) de agua caliente/fría/ hirviendo/tibia	ehn oon KWAHR-toh (PEEN-tah) dai AH-gwah cah-lee-EHN-tai/FREE-ah/ihr-vee-EHN-doh/TIH-bee-ah
with milk	con leche	kon LAI-chai
with juice	con jugo	kon HOO-go
in a glass of water	en un vaso de agua	ehn oon VAH-soh dai AH-gwah

Diseases, Illnesses, and Medical Conditions

English	Spanish	Pronunciation
acne	acné; granos en la cara y espalda	ahk-NAI; GRAH-nos ehn lah CAH-rah ee ehs-PAHL-dah

Diseases, Illnesses, and Medical Conditions

(continued)

English	Spanish	Pronunciation
AIDS	SIDA; síndrome de inmunodeficiencia adquirida	SEE-dah; SIN-droh-mai dai ihn-moo-noh-dai-fee-see-EHN-see-ah ahd-kee-REE-dah
allergy	alergia; reacción a ciertas sustancias	ah-LAIR-hee-ah; rai-ahk-see-OHN ah see-AIR-tas soos-TAHN-see-ahs
anemia	anemia; hemoglobina baja o glóbulos rojos bajos	ah-NAI-mee-ah; hee-moh-gloh-BEE-nah BAH-hah oh GLOH-boo-lohs ROH-hohs BAH-hos
angina	angina	ahn-HEE-nah
arrythmia	arritmia; irregularidad en el pulso	ahr-REET-mee-ah; ih-reh-goo-lah-rih-DAHD ehn ehl POOL-soh
arthritis	artritis; inflamación y dolor en las articulaciones	ahr-TREE-tis; in-flah-mah-see-OHN ee doh-LOHR ehn lahs ahr-tee-koo-lah-see-OH-nais

Diseases, Illnesses, and Medical Conditions

(continued)

English	Spanish	Pronunciation
asthma	asma; súbita falta de aire por inflamación o espasmo de los bronquios	AHS-mah; SOO-bee-tah FAHL-tah dai AI-rai por in-flah-mah-see-OHN oh ehs-PAHS-mo dai lohs BROHN-kee-ohs
blood clot	cuágulo de sangre	koo-AH-goo-loh dai SAHN-grai
bronchitis	bronquitis; inflamación de la mucosa de los bronquios	brohn-KEE-tees; in-flah-mah-see-OHN dai lah moo-KOH-sah dai lohs BROHN-kee-ohs
burn	quemadura	kai-mah-DOO-rah
cancer; cancerous	cáncer; canceroso	KAHN-sair; kahn-sair-ROH-soh
cataract	cataratas	cah-tah-RAH-tahs
chest pain	dolor en el pecho	doh-LOHR ehn ehl PAI-cho
cholecystitis	colecistitis; inflamación de la vesícula	koh-lai-sees-TEE-tis; in-flah-mah-see-OHN dai lah vai-SIH-koo-lah

Diseases, Illnesses, and Medical Conditions

(continued)

English	Spanish	Pronunciation
cholesterol	colesterol	koh-lais-tair-ROHL
cystitis	cistitis; inflamación de la vejiga	sees-TEE-tis; in-flah-mah-see-OHN dai lah veh-HEE-gah
dermatitis	dermatitis; inflamación de la piel	dair-mah-TEE-tis; in-flah-mah-see-OHN dai lah PEE-el
diabetes	diabetes; cantidad abnormal de azúcar en la orina o en la sangre	dee-ah-BAI-tes; kahn-tee-DAHD ahb-nohr-MAHL dai ah-SOO-kahr ehn lah oh-REE-nah oh ehn lah SAHN-grai
dysentery	disentería; desorden intestinal con inflamación de la mucosa	dih-sen-tair-REE-ah; dehs-OR-den in-tehs-tee-NAHL kon in-flah-mah-see-OHN dai lah moo-KOH-sah
eczema	eczema	ehk-SEE-mah
emphysema	enfisema; distensión o ruptura de los alvéolos pulmonales	en-fee-SAI-mah; dihs-tehn-see-OHN oh roop-TOO-rah dai lohs ahl-vai-OH-lohs pool-moh-NAH-lehs

Diseases, Illnesses, and Medical Conditions

(continued)

English	Spanish	Pronunciation
epilepsy	epilepsia; enfermedad asociada con convulsiones	eh-pee-LEHP-see-ah; ehn-fair-meh-DAHD ah-soh-see-AH-dah kon kon-vool-see-OH-nais
fever	fiebre	fee-AI-brai
fracture	fractura	frahk-TOO-rah
gastritis	gastritis; inflamación del estómago	gahs-TREE-tis; in-flah-mah-see-OHN dehl ehs-TOH-mah-go
glaucoma	glaucoma; enfermedad de los ojos con pérdida progresiva de la vista	glau-KOH-mah; en-fair-meh-DAHD dai lohs OH-hohs kon PAIR-dee-dah proh-greh-SEE-vah dai lah VEES-tah
gout	gota	GO-tah
gum disease	enfermedad de las encías	ehn-fair-meh-DAHD dai lahs en-SEE-ahs
hay fever	coriza; rinitis alérgica	koh-REE-sah; ree-NEE-tis ah-LEHR-hee-kah

Diseases, Illnesses, and Medical Conditions

(continued)

English	Spanish	Pronunciation
heart attack	ataque al corazón	ah-TAH-kai ahl koh-rah-SON
heartburn	acidez estomacal; hervedez; ardor de estómago o del esófago	ah-see-DES ehs-toh-mah-KAHL; air-vai-DES; ahr-DOHR dai ehs-TOH-mah-goh oh dehl eh-SOH-fah-goh
hemorrhoids	hemorroides; almorranas; dilatación de los vasos sanguíneos anales	eh-moh-ROI-dais; ahl-mohr-RAH-nahs; dih-lah-tah-see-OHN dai lohs VAH-sos sahn-GEE nai-ohs ah-NAH-lais
hepatitis	hepatitis; inflamación del hígado	eh-pah-TEE-tis; in-flah-mah-see-OHN dehl EE-gah-doh
hives	ronchas; erupción	ROHN-chas; eh-roop-see-OHN
hypertension	hipertensión; presión sanguínea alta	ee-pair-tehn-see-OHN; preh-see-OHN sahn-GEE-nai-ah AHL-tah

Diseases, Illnesses, and Medical Conditions

(continued)

English	Spanish	Pronunciation
hyperthyroidism	hipertiroidismo; niveles altos de las hormonas de la tiroide	ee-pair-tee-roh-ee-DEES-moh; nee-VAI-lais AHL-tohs dai lahs ohr-MOH-nahs dai lah tee-ROI-dai
hypothyroidism	hipotiroidismo; niveles bajos de las hormonas de la tiroide	ee-poh-tee-roh-ee-DEES-moh; nee-VAI-lais BAH-hohs dai lahs ohr-MOH-nahs dai lah tee-ROI-dai
indigestion	indigestión	ihn-dih-hehs-tee-OHN
infected	infectado	ihn-fehk-TAH-doh
infertility	infertilidad	ihn-fair-tee-lee-DAHD
injury	lesión; herida	leh-see-OHN; air-REE-dah
migraine	migraña; jaqueca; dolor severo de cabeza	mee-GRAH-nyah; hah-KAI-kah; doh-LOHR sai-VAI-roh dai kah-BAI-sah

Diseases, Illnesses, and Medical Conditions

(continued)

English	Spanish	Pronunciation
myocardial infarction	infarto al miocardio	ihn-FAHR-toh ahl mee-oh-KAHR-dee-oh
neuralgia	dolor o punzada fuerte en un nervio	doh-LOHR oh puhn-SAH-dah foo-AIR-tai ehn oon NAIR-vee-oh
numbness	adormecimiento	ah-dohr-meh-see-mee-EHN-toh
osteoporosis	osteoporosis	ohs-tee-oh-poh-ROH-sees
otitis	otitis; inflamación del oído interno	oh-TEE-tis; in-flah-mah-see-OHN dehl oh-EE-doh in-TAIR-no
Parkinson's	mal de Parkinson; enfermedad que produce temblores generales	mahl dai pahr-KEEN-sohn; ehn-fair-meh-DAHD kai proh-DOO-sai tehm-BLOH-rais heh-neh-RAH-lais
pneumonia	pulmonía; inflamación de los pulmones	puhl-moh-NEE-ah; in-flah-mah-see-OHN dai lohs puhl-MOH-nais
rash	erupción de la piel	eh-roop-see-OHN dai lah pee-EHL

Diseases, Illnesses, and Medical Conditions

(continued)

English	Spanish	Pronunciation
rhinitis	rinitis; inflamación de la mucosa nasal	ree-NEE-tis; in-flah-mah-see-OHN dai lah moo-KOH-sah nah-SAHL
scarlet fever	fiebre escarlatina	fee-AI-brai ehs-kahr-lah-TEE-nah
schizophrenia/ schizophrenic	esquizofrenia/ esquizofrénico	ehs-kee-soh-FRAI-nee-ah/ehs-kee-soh-FRAI-nee-koh
sinusitis	sinusitis	see-noo-SEE-tis
slipped disc	disco desplazado	DEES-koh dehs-plah-SAH-doh
sprain	torcedura; luxación	tor-seh-DOO-rah; look-sah-see-OHN
tonsillitis	amigdalitis; inflamación de las amígdalas	ah-mihg-dah-LEE-tis; in-flah-mah-see-OHN dai lahs ah-MIHG-dah-lahs

Diseases, Illnesses, and Medical Conditions

(continued)

ulcer

English	Spanish	Pronunciation
peptic ulcer	úlcera péptica	UHL-seh-rah PEP-tee-kah
gastric ulcer	úlcera gástrica	UHL-seh-rah GAHS-tree-kah
duodenal ulcer	úlcera duodenal	UHL-seh-rah doo-oh-dai-NAHL
urine infection	infección de la orina	ihn-fehk-see-OHN dai lah ohr-REE-nah

Drug Classes

English	Spanish	Pronunciation
analgesic	analgésico; calmante para el dolor	ah-nahl-HEH-see-koh; kahl-MAHN-tai PAH-rah ehl doh-LOHR
anesthetic	anestésico	ah-nais-TEH-see-koh
antacid	antiácido	ahn-tee-AH-see-doh
antibiotic	antibiótico	ahn-tee-bee-OH-tee-koh

Drug Classes (continued)

English	Spanish	Pronunciation
anticoagulant	anticoagulante	ahn-tee-koh-ah-goo-LAHN-tai
antihistaminic	antihistamínico	ahn-tee-ihs-tah-MEE-nee-koh
anti-inflammatory	antiinflamatorio	ahn-tee-ihn-flah-mah-TOH-ree-oh
antiseptic	antiséptico	ahn-tee-SEP-tee-koh
barbiturate	barbitúrico	bahr-bee-TOO-ree-koh
chemotherapy	quimioterapia	kee-mee-oh-tair-RAH-pee-ah
contraceptive	contraceptivo	kohn-trah-sep-TEE-voh
cough drops	pastillas para la tos	pahs-TEE-yahs PAH-rah lah tohs
diuretic	diurético; agente que aumenta la cantidad de orina	dee-oo-REH-tee-koh; ah-HEN-tai kai au-MEN-tah lah kahn-tee-DAHD dai ohr-REE-nah
immunosuppressants	inmunosupresores	ihn-moo-noh-soo-prai-SOH-rais

Drug Classes (continued)

English	Spanish	Pronunciation
insulin	insulina	ihn-soo-LEE-nah
laxative	laxante	lahk-SAN-tai
narcotics	narcótico	nahr-KOH-tee-koh
nutritional supplements	suplementos nutricionales	soo-plai-MEN-tohs noo-tree-see-oh-NAH-lais
sedative	sedativo; sedante	seh-dah-TEE-vo; seh-DAHN-tai
steroid	esteroide	ehs-tair-ROEE-dai
tranquilizer	calmante para los nervios	kahl-MAHN-tai PAH-rah los NAIR-vee-ohs
vaccine	vacuna	vah-KOO-nah
vitamins	vitaminas	vee-tah-MEE-nahs

Other Pharmacy Terms

English	Spanish	Pronunciation
contraindications	contraindicaciones	kon-tra-ihn-dee-kah-see-OH-nais
disease	enfermedad	ehn-fair-meh-DAHD
dose	la dosis	lah DOH-sees
expiration date	fecha de expiración	FAI-cha dai ehk-spee-rah see-OHN
habit forming	puede causar hábito	PWAI-dai kau-SAHR AH-bee-toh
pharmacist/patient interaction	interacción farmacéutico/ paciente	in-tair-ahk-see-OHN fahr-mah-see-OO-tee-koh/pah-see-EN-tai
sick	enfermo	ehn-FAIR-moh
side effects	efectos adversos	eh-FEHK-tohs ahd-VAIR-sohs

Pronunciation Guide

Pronunciation Guide

Letter	Sounds Like	Sample Spanish Word
a	"a" in "father"	cama (bed) = KAH-mah
b	"b" in "bed"	boca (mouth) = BOH-kah
c	"k" as in "cut" unless before "e" or "i"	cuello (neck) = KWAI-yoh
c	"s" as in "medicine" when before "e" or "i"	medicina (medicine) = meh-dee-SEE-nah
ch	"ch" in "church"	mucho (a lot) = MOO-choh
d	"d" in "dirt"	diarrea (diarrhea) = dee-ah-RAI-ah
e	"e" in "wet"	pecho (chest) = PAI-choh
f	"f" in "family"	fiebre (fever) = fee-AI-brai
g	"g" in "good" unless before "e" or "i"	garganta (throat) = gahr-GAN-tah
g	"h" in "help" when before "e" and "i"	alergia (allergy) = ah-LAIR-hee-ah
h	*silent*	hospital (hospital) = ohs-pee-TAHL
i	"ee" in "seen" but a bit shorter	inyecte (inject) = ihn-YEHK-tai
j	"h" in "home"	ojo (eye) = OH-ho
k	"k" in "kite"	kilo (kilo) = KEE-loh
l	"l" in "long"	lengua (tongue) = LAING-gwah
ll	"y" in "yes"	tobillo (ankle) = toh-BEE-yoh
m	"m" in "man"	mano (hand) = MAH-noh

Letter	Sounds Like	Sample Spanish Word
n	"n" in nothing"	nariz (nose) = nah-REES
ñ	"ni" in "onion"	riñón (kidney) = ree-NYON
o	"o" in know	codo (elbow) = KOH-doh
p	"p" in pear	pantorrilla (calf) = pahn-toh-REE-yah
qu	"k" in "kick" (u is silent)	esquizofrenia (schizophrenia) = ehs-kee-soh-FRAI-nee-ah
r	soft rolled r	rodilla (knee) = rho-DEE-yah
rr	hard rolled r	catarro (cold) = kah-TAH-rhoh
s	"s" in "solid"	senos (breasts) = SAI-nohs
t	"t" in "toe" but tongue is placed closer to teeth	tres (three) = TRAIS
u	"oo" in "food"	diluya (dilute) = dee-LOO-yah
u	"w" (usually) when followed by vowel	duerme (sleep) = DWAIR-mai
u	*silent after "q" or in "gue" and "gui"*	quemadura (burn) = kai-mah-DOO-rah
v	"b" in "but"	vena (vein) = VAI-nah
x	"x" in "maximum"	laxante (laxative) = lahk-SAN-tai
y	"y" in "yes"	yeso (cast) = yeh-SOH
z	"s" in "sun"	corazón (heart) = koh-rah-SOHN
z	"s" in "six"	zapatos (shoes) = sah-PAH-tohs